Contents

For Complete Beginners – What is Cholinergic Urticaria

The NHS describes Urticaria as a condition which occurs when histamine and other chemicals are released from under the skin's surface, causing the tissues to swell[i]. Urticaria is commonly know as hives, which is a reaction most suffers get to the release of histamine and other chemicals. Cholinergic urticaria is a form of urticaria which is usually triggered by sweat related events, including but not limited to exercise, stress and heat.

The symptoms are usually an intense itching feeling followed by an outbreak of redness in the inflamed areas, and usually with physical hives (lumps) on the skin. The sufferers normally feel like "burning up" as the reaction is happening.

For me personally the stages felt as follows:

1. Feeling of warmth out of nowhere, particularly around my arms, face and hair (Hair usually first but not always).
2. Tense feeling as heat builds
3. Quickly followed with hives outbreak and redness/red spots. Typically hives on my arms, chest and back, while red spots on my forehead.
4. Severe itchy skin for 5-10 minutes.
5. Itching dies down but hives remain for another 10-20 minutes

NOTE: If the outbreak was minor it is easily triggered again within a ten minute period. Major outbreaks send to "reset the counter".

The itching for me comes along mostly just before I am going to sweat. For example, I am doing something which is warming up my body but not enough for any major exertion. Some people only get this feeling or a breakout during exercise, and it can be called exercise urticaria. However as you will find out, that is not the case for me and thousands of other sufferers.

I will go into this in more detail, but a simple way of thinking about urticaria and the build up to itching is you have a jug with a tiny hole in the bottom. As you do things that exert you or cause you stress, the tap turns on and the jug gets more water in it. The more intense the trigger the faster the water fills the jug. If you stop for a while, the water can drain out slowly through the tiny hole at the bottom, however if one drip overflows out of the top, you will have a break out.

What An Attack Can Look Like

Here are various examples of myself with hives. As you can see the look of it can change quite dramatically depending on severity.

Image 1 – An average amount of hives on my arm. The itching is still felt all over, despite the lack of redness or particularly large number of hives

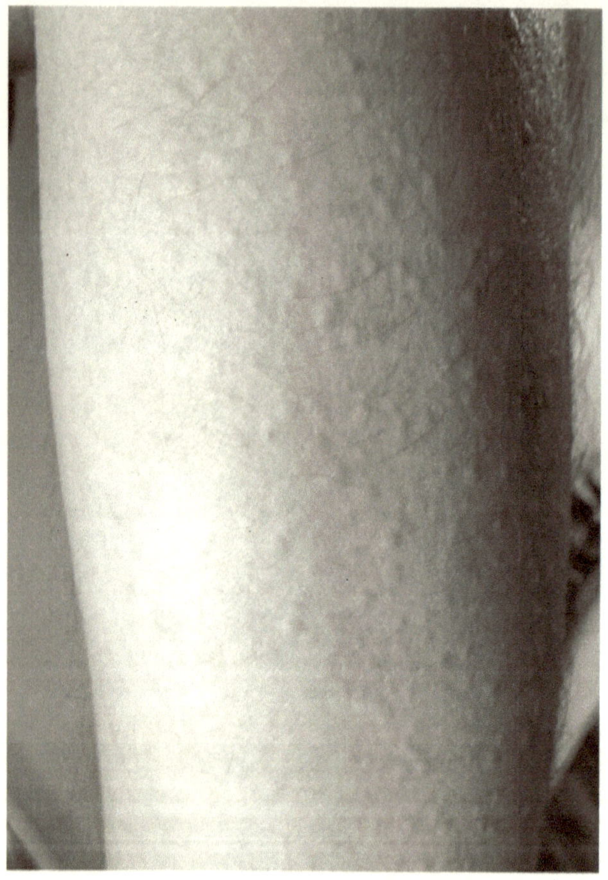

Image 2 – Large number of hives on my back. You can clearly see the clusters.

Image 3 – Redness on back (may not show up clearly on black and white Kindle devices) and covered with hives

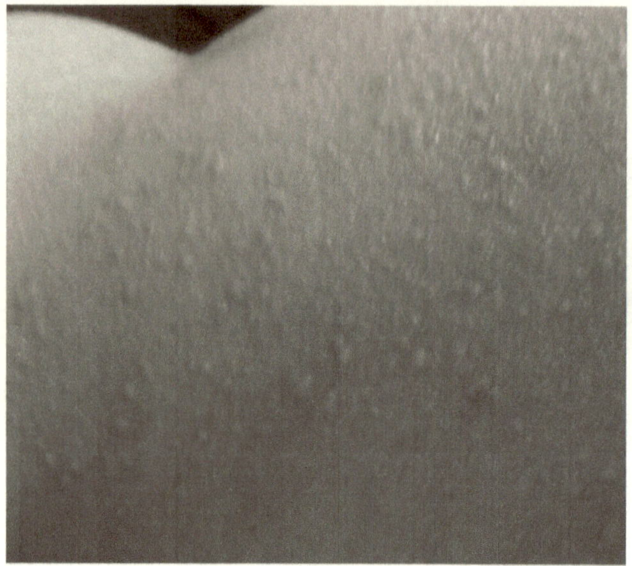

Where I Was At To How I Am Now

My cholinergic urticaria started in the summertime, when I initially passed it off for letting my hair get too long (not long long, just long for me) and my head being itchy because it was too warm. However one hair cut later and within a month I got my first bad itching and redness with hives when at the gym. This was all over my arms and in my hairline, so clearly not exclusively to do with heat in my head.

This lead to a two year plus period of urticaria running and ruining my life. A simple short walk to a friends or the local shops became something I had to plan in advance and usually ended in agony. I could not exercise at all, and had to quit the gym I was attending. This caused me to drive everywhere, which had its own set of problems. In summer, if the car was hot as I got into it, attack. Whilst driving if someone brakes sharply making me "jump", or does something stupid and unexpected, itching starts.

Winters were particularly bad. Going into town, all the shops and restaurants had the heating on maximum, and this resulted in my average shop visit being about 30 seconds to 1 minute. And the few shops that I could stand, I felt like I couldn't speak to a member of staff for fear of an attack, which happened many times. When the weather was particularly bad, and snow and ice were around, it made walking unbearable. Every slip, however minor seemed to jolt my body which caused the feeling of an itch coming.

Food was a particularly bad area that got me down. I love my food, but I couldn't eat a single hot meal at home or in a restaurant without an attack for a long period. Want to eat that meal that you have always loved, attack! It regularly got so bad that I had to strip off and jump in the shower to calm it down on many occasions. Multiple trips to the dermatologist and doctor with literally hundreds of tablets taken in a short period of time, and nothing had improved.

However I am happy to say that although my urticaria has not gone completely, it no longer rules my life. I do, see, and eat what I want. No longer is going to the shops or a friends house a worrying prospect. I am reasonably fit again and I have taken maybe 3 antihistamine tablets in the last year. I can't actually remember the last time I had a bad hives attack, and I believe I can keep it this way.

What changed for me was I began measuring my triggers, attacks, and changed my mindset towards the condition. Some of this is easier said than done, but if you can work out what it is that sets you off the most, and change how you view it I believe you can really change how urticaria affects your life. First, lets look at triggers.

Triggers

There are many triggers to my Cholinergic Urticaria. However everyone has their own main triggers, and other smaller ones unique to them. Some of which can be hard to define, as the primary culprit is not always obvious. This following list of triggers may also give you some ideas of what it is that sets you off, as some of you may not have worked out exactly what it is that causes your urticaria outbreaks.

It took me a long time, months, to single out the different causes. In many cases it can appear to be one thing, when the underlying issue is something else unexpected. There are some things I have found that cause a reaction faster which are quite surprising and contradictory to the basic principles of "I'm hot, cool down as quick as you can!"

Food & Eating

The first thing that comes to mind with food and bad reactions is allergies. I have no history of allergies, but I have personally known people who have had allergies come on for several months to certain types of food, to only die down again, so I thought it could be an issue. However my Dermatologist said there is "very little point" in doing allergy testing for urticaria as they produce too may false positives. I felt this was true as even with some of my worst foods for setting me off, I could eat a small amount of any without issue. Listed below in this section are food items listed that I have had a reaction with over the past couple of years.

What do I class as "urticaria reaction"? Itching to the extent I have hives, or have to leave the room due to heat while trying not to itch or while itching.

Food is a large issue for most cholinergic urticaria sufferers. There are multiple aspects of food, and eating situations which can cause itching. There are numerous theories dermatologists, fellow sufferers and myself have found to be triggers. The food itself, types of ingredients, the way it is cooked, location you are eating in, environmental factors (heat in room etc.), even who you are eating with can all play a large part in what sets you off. As with so many cholinergic urticaria triggers, it is a personal thing as to what sets you off. Try to find patterns and make a note of these factors and you should be able to cut back on attacks.

Note on my preferences / diet:
As I said I have zero known food allergies before my urticaria or even now. And as previous mentioned my Dermatologist told me food allergy tests give up too many false positives to be worth while. I used to eat what I wanted to quiet liberally. I have always had a balanced diet of healthy food, with a leaning towards spicy and Asian influenced foods as my favourites. I am a healthy man of average build, and have no dietary or weight problems.

Your Eating Environment:

One of the biggest problems for a CU sufferer is eating. However sometimes it is not the food that is the problem. Your eating environment can be a major trigger for the itching to start. When I say environment, these are the factors which are not directly related to the food on your plate, but the place you are in and the company you are with. One of the most overlooked factors is where you eat. Everyday triggers like heat change, stress, excitement, and anxiety all can play a factor when eating a meal, so where you eat can make a difference to all of these symptoms.

Eating At Home

Despite being in the comfort of your own home, meal time can become a nightmare for itching. I have had several periods where literally every hot meal was a cause of a urticaria outbreak. I mostly have this under control now, and I have managed to do this, via a process of elimination and working out patterns. The result of this is actually quite simple. Although it won't necessarily be the same for you, hence why I recommend trying the different environmental changes I have done, and make a note of the times they help. Even if help means, your itching dies down quicker rather than getting rid of it completely. If it doesn't come up at all, then great but you and I know this is not always possible.

The most significant change for me is to try to keep the room as cool as possible while cooking, e.g. make sure you have windows open, and doors if possible. Keep them open while you eat also. Although this will not dramatically change the temperature after the initial drop, it does help create a breeze and reduces the residual heat in the room from the oven or stoves, which for me creates a more relaxing dining experience. If your house is open plan and you have been cooking for 30 minutes, that heat can stay in the room for a surprisingly long time, by reducing this as much as possible really helped me. Its a small change but one I have found time and time again to really help, even if that is just a mental thing. Being in your own home allows you to control environmental factors, which means you can then test food in a more controlled environment with less variables. So once you can control your eating environment somewhat, you can then get onto the food itself.

Eating out at a restaurant

To start with, you have no control over the temperature of the restaurant, except to maybe sit near a window if available. Temperature shock (coming in from the cold to a baking hot restaurant/shop) on its own has been enough to set me off with really bad hives. Now if you are out at a restaurant chances are you are there for an occasion, a party, a date, or even just a catch up with friends. Each of these situations offer up a different area to set you off on an attack, such as stress, eustress or excitement. And this is before the food is even on the table, and who knows what triggers that might set off! So how can we ease these symptoms when there is no where to go, and no shower to jump into? First thing is be prepared. If you mentally prepare for the restaurant to be hot, and take off your coat and jumper etc as soon as you get it, in your mind you are ready to be as cool as you can, just incase. With heat related urticaria triggers, you can never be too cold! Once you get used to the temperature of the restaurant, if you decide you are a bit cold you can add a layer back on. If you are like me, you will probably be hot most of the time this will not be an issue.

What about the excitement or anxiety of being around people, and being up close and personal in a crowded environment? This is a tough one, although I find it easier, if possible, to arrange to meet on the way rather than straight at the restaurant. This allows you to deal with one thing at a time. You can do the meet and greet, then deal with the restaurant (temperature etc., as described above), and then the food. However this is not always possible. It is not something you can always control, however you can still take it in stages, you just have to modify how you do it.

One of my favourite ways when I was really bad was to say hello, take your coat off etc., but then excuse yourself to the toilet. It is a completely natural thing to do, so there is nothing to worry about what people might think. You can then take some time out, relax if you are feeling the urticaria bubbling up, and then come back and say your hello's properly. The more you can break up the stages in your mind, the more relaxed and in control you feel. Despite all these techniques being related to the hives and itching, you find that you are thinking less, "please don't itch!" as you are concentrating on the solutions to make it better. Accept the fact it will not get rid of it totally, but also accept that you are going through the steps to make it less extreme for you.

Now you just have to order! I wont go over specific foods, as I mention them in this section, however with restaurant food, try to think how the food will be presented. Is it going to be on a sizzling hot plate which will blow hot steam all over my personal space, or is it something mega spicy that will have me worried, or worse people talking about my food! I am not saying do not eat what you want, just judge how you are feeling in the environment at the time and go from there. If you are struggling, then try to avoid (or limit if the menu does not allow it) your known trigger foods.

One more thing on restaurants, I personally have noticed that if going out in a group rather than just a small number like four people, I tend to find my itching is dramatically reduced. The above techniques for restaurants also works if you are invited for a meal at someone else's house.

Testing For What Sets You Off

Before I get onto what foods have caused me a reaction, I wanted to talk about how to test for triggers. When doing any experimentation it is important to get the variables which are not being tested as close to the "norm" as possible. The variable we are testing is the food itself. This means don't eat a pizza at home, and then at a restaurant and make a decision that pizza sets you off and you should never eat it again. All food testing should be done in a place where environmental conditions are as similar as possible. This usually means at home. Next, get comfortable, open a window while cooking and eating if required to get a somewhat stable temperature. Eat in light comfortable clothing, e.g. a T-Shirt or light top. What we are trying to do is eliminate as many of the other environmental factors/triggers as possible. Once this has been achieved try out differences to see what sets you off.

The Pasta Example

I am a pasta lover and I found several times that I would get attacks eating things like Spaghetti Bolognese and my personal favourite, Meatballs in Arrabiata. Because most pastas are relatively simple dishes, they are ideal for trialling different product variations.

There was nothing fancy to this at the beginning. I first tried different brands of sauces, then different ingredients (mince, Quorn, chicken, vegetable), pasta types (brands, wholewheat, shape) etc. etc. Each meal had one variation of ingredient. This testing allowed me to find out that green pesto based dishes did not set me off. I could repeat this several times, and have no or very little reaction. Whereas almost every time a store bought tomato based pasta sauce (the famous UK brands everyone knows) would set me off. At this time I was convinced it was something in tomato based sauces that was a bad trigger for me. Tomato based curry sauces were also a bad trigger. Then by chance I tried a home-made recipe and did not have as much of a reaction! I made it with a simple tin of chopped tomatoes, garlic, mixed herbs, red wine, salt and pepper, and it was fine. Great but I understand it can be quite a lot of effort for some people everytime you want a quick pasta dish. So I then tried a packet mix for bolognese, where you mix a packet with a tin of chopped tomatoes, and added some red wine for extra flavour. Firstly it tasted great, much better than the jar versions, but it also does not set me off! Strike up another dish for back on my menu!

Will this be the same for you, no, but if you can make small changes to your favourite dishes you may see an improvement which will allow you to pick out what it is that has made the difference. Almost universally homemade always seems to improve things, but I understand for some people it is not always viable. But the more natural the better! However random simple things like packet mixes have made a large difference to me. Looking at the ingredients, it is impossible for me to say what the trigger ingredient is, but there must be something in the process of how it is made that uses less ingredients which I believe helps.

Below are a list of foods / condiments which I have had a reaction to on a regular basis, and the variations that I have tried. As I said, I went for a period of a couple of months where almost every meal I had set me off. However all of these have consistently caused itching or hives on multiple occasions in the same environment (at home).

Tomato Based Pasta Sauces – Shop bought ones tend to cause a worse reaction than homemade ones. E.g. Bolognese sauce, chunky or smooth. To get less of a reaction but still enjoy one of my favourite foods I have found packet mixes, where you add chopped tomatoes and red wine to the sauce, cause less of a reaction. The type of pasta (wholewheat or white) seems to make no difference. Brand of pasta also makes no difference.

Curry Sauces (Indian and Thai) – Spicier sauces bring out the fastest reaction. However even mild curries eventually do. I used to be a "heat seaker" and had hot sauce on everything, so I have no history of problems with heat. I do not find 90% of the curries I eat hot that make me break out, but it makes no difference to the itching. I eat the curries always with white rice, and sometimes with naan bread. I found some improvement with wholegrain rice and again homemade sauces were much better.

Hot Sauces – My downfall, as I love hot sauce on everything from toast to pizza! Heat of the sauce however is irrelevant to the amount of itching. In my testing pepper type has seen a noticeable trend. Scotch Bonnet based sauces, which tend to be West Indian sauces like Encona, Dunns River etc. are better for itching than Indian / Thai based sauces. If you are a huge hot sauce fan like me and still find it difficult, then all you can do is compromise. Either get rid of your hot sauces, a painful moment for any heat seeker, or mix! In recent times I have found if I mix Encona Hot Pepper Sauce (my favourite) with another sauce (BBQ for example), it not only tastes delicious, but it doesn't set me off as easily. Try mixing to not only dilute the spice, but create a new blend which goes well with a wide variety of dishes.

Vinegars (Malt and Balsamic) – I love vinegar on chips, and balsamic vinegar on salads. These do not cause a major reaction but noteworthy. Hair itching is a regular occurrence if I go a bit over the top with the vinegar. If the food I have eaten is "neutral" then this is normally OK, but if I was borderline itching before, it can send it over the edge.

Other Diets Tried:
My dermatologist put me on an almost paleo diet, where I was asked to not eat anything processed, or any red meats. The idea here was to break down my food intake into the most basic forms. I was given a huge list which consisted of basically every food I liked and told not to eat it. All I had were standard British vegetables like potatoes, peas, broccoli, sweetcorn, with white meats – chicken, pork, and fish. I had to avoid tomatoes, tomato based products, lots of condiments, even things orange juice. This diet did help with my food based attacks, they became less frequent and intense, but it did not help with exercise or stress related flare ups. My main problem with the diet was that I began to become bored with eating, which for a large foodie like myself was not a nice place to be. Although it did help me confirm a few pointers about how non processed foods and sauces definitely make a positive difference. This led me to discoveries confirming how homemade foods created less itching, while having a meal that I actually wanted to eat. In the end after 6 weeks of hardcore boredom eating, I incorporated it into my everyday meals once a week, or more if I had had a bad day.

One Final Comment on Low Histamine Diets:
I have read about and trialled low histamine diets. The theory makes sense,

eat foods that are naturally low in histamine would mean less attacks. It did not make any difference to me over a two month trial period, but looking at what you eat and making patterns in what does and more crucially, what does *not* set you off could make your life much better! This is what I hoped to achieve.

Exercise:

One of the biggest issues with urticaria for me and a lot of people is that it makes exercise very difficult at best, and impossible at worst. There is nothing worst than the feeling of doing very minor exercise, something which you used to not even think about, but now it makes you want to rip your skin off as it makes you feel immensely uncomfortable. It is always just before you are about to sweat that the itching would come. If on the rare occasion that I could fight through it and actually sweat, it would go. However this is rarely possible when you are having a particularly bad time. When this was at its worst, I had to make sure my diet was good as I knew I wouldn't be able to burn off those calories. Even today I am nowhere near as fit as I want to be as I cannot exert myself how I want. However I have found ways to build up tolerance to return to some level of fitness. Below are some of the forms of exercise which have regularly set me off.

Walking for greater than 10 minutes – Probably the most frustrating trigger. This means sometimes I choose not to go places as I don't want to scratch all over and feel uncomfortable. I have missed out on a lot of things because of this. Again it comes on without me feeling hot or out of breathe. I am talking about very minor exercise.

Walking Up Hills, Even Small Hills – This is a killer every time. The strange part about this, is I start itching near the bottom of the hill, so its not as though its been brought on by getting out of breathe. Maybe this is due to the thought of "this is going to make me itch" or it has in the past and I am bringing the association of this with it.

The Gym – I had to quit my gym membership as it was one of the places I first noticed the itching come up. The gym I went to was normally warm, which does not help, but it seems certain exercises set it off more than others. Rowing machine was fine for example, however the seated bench press and the pull down row almost instantly brought on the itching. I tended to do higher weights (for me), which the strain seems to set it off. However I can tend to do bicep curls for as long as I physically can with no itching, so I feel maybe there is a particular movement issue, but I have not been able to work out what that movement is due to the equipment I have available to me.

Cycling – Cycling is an odd one, as again it tends to trigger at similar moments to walking, e.g. going up hills. Also, similar to walking there seems to be a limit in distance I can take until the itching comes. Usually the itching starts in my hair, and then spreads to chest, back and arms. Ambient temperature does not seem to matter, although oddly I have found wearing a t-shirt and having exposed arms makes it MORE susceptible to itching than a long sleeve, which was surprising as the wind can not cool your arms down. This happens repeatedly in similar temperatures. Try this out and see if this is the same for you.

Swimming – Pools are usually cooler, which allow me to do more exercise. However I have had mild to medium reactions if I try to push it and do some fast lengths. This can create a weird feeling of itching whilst being in cool water. But overall swimming is one of the ways I would recommend for keeping your fitness. I had the opposite effect at the Blue Lagoon in Iceland, where the water was 30oC but above water was -5oC. There it was a case of feel the itch, stand up! Gone in seconds. Great for hot baths and spas. Steam rooms I found to be easier to stay in than saunas, probably due to the immense humidity, but I can not relax properly in either when the urticaria was really bad.

Notes on Being Fit and Returning to a Fitness:

Like many urticaria suffers, my fitness levels dropped dramatically due to not being able to do exercise comfortably. While I am not going to do the Marathon des Sables anytime soon, I feel that I once again have a decent level of fitness. I achieved this by doing small, sometimes ridiculously small, steps to gain the fitness back. It is hard to be disciplined to not go too far, but if you can build up, you will be surprised by how far you can eventually go. I was lucky enough to have a friend who is a keen runner come out with me. I cycled while he ran (I hate running and besides could never keep up with him anyway, he actually has done the Marathon des Sables!). We started off by doing short distances for him, but a challenge for me (3 mile loop), and within a month progressed to 8 mile loops. Since I have done over 10 miles in a morning regularly with minimal or even no itching which never fails to put a smile on my face. I was never tired after the shorter loops, but I know that the itching was just around the next corner if I went another mile. I think building up your fitness is a great physiological way to reduce urticaria. Like previously mentioned, there will be some movements you will not be able to do easily, so you will have to adjust for what works. For me this was cycling arms covered, and doing press ups/squats. Psychologically having someone chatting to me, and talking to them, whilst cycling around sometimes picturesque places really helped to take the mind off the potential situation. When by myself I find listening to podcasts or non-fiction audio-books rather than music is better for this. Plus you may actually learn something and take information in, rather than just listening to songs which may let the mind wander to other urticaria related areas!

Anxiety Related:

This is something new to me which I found out (the hard way), and I can not explain it as being anything other than anxiety related urticaria. I walked home from a friends house less than 5 minutes away and I could see down the road (around 100 metres away) someone emptying their car of shopping, going in and out of their house. I thought nothing of it, and in a nice friendly manner, as I approached close to their car they said "Hello" and proceeded to go inside. I replied "Hi" and within seconds I had a major itching breakout which lead to hives. This caused me to connect anxiety as a major trigger to my urticaria. I am traditionally, and even now, not an anxious person or someone who suffers from anxiety in any none urticaria form. I normally have no problems talking to people or being exposed to new situations etc. However I do not see what else that could have been. It also matches up with some previous experiences, like in shops worrying about an outbreak if I have to talk to a member of staff. Or something/someone you weren't expecting in a situation, or having to talk to someone you haven't met before. These have proved to be triggers for me, and maybe for you without realising it.

In many ways the fear of breaking out itching in a social situation is one of the biggest problems facing urticaria sufferers. It is a vicious circle as you can experience anxiety worrying about a break out, but worrying about it will most likely make you break out.

In and out of Shops:

Particularly in Winter this is a "killer" trigger for me. Its cold outside and you are wrapped up, comfortably warm. Then you go into a shop and they have the heating on full whack so the staff can walk around in t-shirts while its freezing outside. I have had to literally run out of shops due to the oncoming feeling. 30 seconds is my "best" in one particular high street store before having to bail. Not only is the heat an issue, but there is the anxiety related problems with staff, as previous mentioned as well as being around lots of people in a confined area.

Shops can be a tough environment when you are struggling. Similar to a busy restaurant, there can be so much going on at once which can be overwhelming. This is why you have to try and change your mindset on how you view the experience.

Showering, Specifically Coming out of the Shower:

I love my long warm showers. However too long and they can set off the beginnings of itching. Sometimes when shampooing at the end of a shower can cause me to want to get out a bit quicker than I would like. When my urticaria was at its worst, the major trigger was getting out of the shower. Going from the warm steam and water to the cool air, and then warming up the skin with the drying would cause a reaction. Soothing creams, such as cocoa butter and other moisturisers help cool the urticaria down, but do not always work.

Reluctantly lowering the temperature of the shower certainly has helped, as has having shorter showers. One proven method for me is having the last minute of the shower near cold. This not only lowers your body temperature, but also reduces steam in the room and prepares you for outside the shower. Cold showers are crazy talk for crazy people I know! But if you can put up with it, it helps. A less painful way is getting out of the shower room after a quick pat down and dry off in a different room. If that's not possible try just opening the door for a few seconds to let the steam out.

A drying tip, try patting in the areas prone to itching rather than rubbing with the towel. Rubbing skin dry will only aggravate things. It takes a little longer, but the time you lose by drying slower using this technique will be gained back from time saved from trying not to scratch or not having an attack!

What I've Taken / Things That Helped

As with many of you I have been given a huge cocktail of drugs to take over the years. From tablets one a day to four a day, and I'm sure some people have been told to take more! As of the last six months I have been "clean" of all tablets, and only in the last 12 months have I had a few times where I reached for the antihistamines. Below I will explain where and what I was given, and my review of each for its overall effects, and how they helped (where applicable). Please consult your doctor before taking any of these. I am not a doctor in anyway, just a patient describing my conditions! Different tablets work for different people.

My aim of this section is to show you the vast array of options for treatment out there, with the hope that they can help you identify what is out there, with the goal of not needing to take anything and just enjoying life again!

Antihistamines

My old friend and enemy, and probably yours too. Anyone who has been to a Doctor or Dermatologist for cholinergic urticaria has been prescribed some sort of antihistamines. Personally I started on a one a day Cetirizine tablet with the option of taking a second if an attack occurred. They had no effect on my urticaria. They did not make it any less frequent or intense. As zero of an effect as possible. Next up was Fexofenadine 180mg. Again nothing. Levocetirizine was prescribed from the dermatologist and I was told to take up to four a day for a period. I was also told to take one before exercise if I knew I was going to go to the gym etc. There was no difference in time or intensity of the attack coming on, whether taking it immediately before, 30 minutes before or just earlier in the day.

With these I noticed no improvement despite this massive dosages being taken, so I stopped. You do not need to be a doctor to realise taking four tablets a day for two months will give side effects, especially when the box says one a day. I could deal with that if they helped, but they did not. I consistently felt tired and lethargic, possibly due to the stress of the attacks and the seemingly nothing I could do about them. The best antihistamine tablet for me was Loratadine 10mg, which I bought on a whim from an online chemist for really cheap. I was incredibly surprised at its calming affects when having an attack. It did not prevent an outbreak but when they came, it calmed them down quicker than any other antihistamine I took. When I told the dermatologist they were not surprised and said that each person's body is unique in how it deals with antihistamines. Some work better for others, much like how different people get different triggers. It was nice to know that I could finally carry something in my wallet which I know would actually help when the attack came, even if it could not stop it in the first place. I bought a basic "non branded" version of the antihistamine. There is no need to get the branded £5 a box version of a tablet you can get for a tenth of the price, especially when you are taking them in these quantities.

If you are having no luck with your current antihistamine, try one of the types I have mentioned above. One make work for you like Loratadine did for me.

But better than that, if you can kick the antihistamines you will be really happy in more than one way. For months I never left the house without some form of antihistamine in my wallet or bag. The frustration of being an otherwise healthy person having to suddenly take these tablets which did not even stop what I was taking them for, despite massive dosages, was beyond annoying. However the backlog I bought is now proudly in the cupboard rarely being used. Using this cocktail of antihistamines with little effect lead me to trying alternative routes, like acupuncture, which I will talk about later.

Supplements – Particularly Magnesium

There is a large dark area over the benefits of vitamins and supplements for urticaria. Lots of people on forums claim Magnesium tablets and general vitamins can dramatically reduce the symptoms of urticaria. Although there is no medical evidence to suggest low magnesium can help make urticaria worse or more frequently triggered, many people swear by it particularly Magnesium Citrate.

Why Citrates, well they are quickly absorbed into the blood stream. One of the benefits of taking Magnesium Citrates, as said on my Holland & Barrett bottle is "Magnesium contributes to the normal functioning of the nervous system" and "supports normal neurotransmission and muscle contraction." In theory this sounds like something most urticaria suffers can relate too and could potentially be beneficial. As previous mentioned, stressful situations are one of my prime triggers in particular. If an imbalance in the nervous system has caused this by sending too much histamine, then all is solved.

Unfortunately I did not see a night and day difference. Mentally I felt the few days I did not take the three a day capsules I had a bad day, however I had bad days with them so I did not see a cause and effect or even a correlation. I went through three bottles, enough for 90 days, with no significant improvement, but I'm sure it did great for my bones and teeth. But going back to other suffers experiences, some people swear by magnesium as an effective way of helping with the intensity of the itching or outbreak full stop. At around £6 for a bottle in the UK (and normally on offer 3 for 2), its an inexpensive trial that might work for you. Foods that are rich in magnesium include almond butter, flaxseed, pumpkin seeds, and unsweetened cocoa, so you may also want to try these for a less chalky way of taking magnesium. You can get them in most whole food stores.

Glorious Copenhagen & Acupuncture

Copenhagen is one of the best places I have travelled to, however this is not a travel journal so why am I mentioning it? Well, in the weeks coming up to my trip I was very worried that it would be ruined by my urticaria. The previous weeks had been horrible as we had had a few nice days here in the UK, so it was a struggle going out and about, something you always want to do on holiday! The Copenhagen temperature was looking mid to high 20s (Celsius) so it was a genuine concern that I would be constantly in agony.

Just a couple of weeks before I was in the height of my tablet regime and was fed up of no results. I thought I may as well not take them! So I looked up alternative therapies and saw that the local University did acupuncture. Now I really hate the idea of such a thing, but surely its worth a try since traditional Western medicine has not helped at all, bar sometimes calming it down once an attack has already ruined whatever it was I was doing. I nervously went along for my first session, and was treated with just four needles (a gentle introduction). This was the end of the week before leaving for Denmark. I took my Loratadine with me, however in a one week holiday of constant walking, warm weather, new experiences, I only had one attack, and it was only minor! I could not believe it. The itching took a few weeks to come back, and I went back to acupuncture really looking forward (as much as you can look forward to someone sticking needles in your head, arms and legs) to more treatment. After years of nothing working, this had calmed it down! And virtually overnight. Maybe there was a bit of being comfortable and loving the Danish sights, however it had had an effect and I wanted more. This was a turning point.

If you are now waiting for me to proclaim alternative medicine, and specially acupuncture as the total solution to urticaria, it's not. But over time I stuck with it for nearly a year, and within months I saw significant consistent reduction in my symptoms. My maximum pain/itching from an attack also lowered from a 10 to a 7, and that is a victory in itself, nevermind the fact that I got less frequent attacks as my threshold for the itching to start had increased. Normally it took a day or two after a treatment session for me to see a significant benefit. However this would then last several weeks before the urticaria started to come back. My optimum time between treatments for "top ups" was three weeks. If I left it four weeks I tended to start seeing the beginnings of a bad week, while two weeks did not seem to make much difference and obviously increased the cost.

My experience with acupuncture was very good, but difficult at times. In the beginning I was very nervous about having needles stuck in me, and once in some needles would set off my urticaria. In fact most did, especially at the beginning. However I was reassured by the specialists that this was a good thing as it was "allowing the pressure to release". Plus you will not scratch the itch when you have needles sticking in you which can hurt if you move too much!

Turns out they were right about the pressure release theory. Although on the day after the acupuncture I did not see the benefit, over the coming week I would always see a great difference in how I felt. I would take those few moments of being uncomfortable in exchange for a couple weeks of reduced itching any day! In fact during the treatment once the needles are in and you have settled down, if I had an initial reaction which was not always the case, it is quite relaxing actually. You are normally left for 15-20 minutes in a quiet room and you can really relax. Because you are lying or sitting very still it is quite meditative and personally it felt like the heat was gently releasing out of the points.

The whole process is genuinely reassuring. Unlike at a Doctor's surgery where you are in and out before you know it, you sit down and talk about what triggers you have, how your condition has been since the last treatment, your diet, feelings, improvements/changes since last session, even bowel movements! You get the sense that they actually are interested in helping find a solution which, again is very reassuring rather than just pumping you out for the next patient due to time constraints.

For those interested and want to try it, the aim for my acupuncture was to reduce my body heat. In Chinese medicine some people are naturally warm (like me), while some are cool. The diagnoses from the specialist was that my energy flow gets stuck and heat is trapped in me which eventually causes the outbreaks. If you want to visit someone who does acupuncture my main points were Gb 20, Du 20, Li11, Sj 6. Give it a try, I cannot recommend it enough. Expect it to itch a bit when the needles initially go in, but a good acupuncture practitioner will take it slow and allow you to cool down and go at your own pace. A massive thank you to Lisa from the University of Lincoln Health Centre for the information, the support and for putting up with me really not liking the needles at times! I would not be in the position I am without the help.

Tools To Help

Lots of people get caught up with fancy tools and apps that do lots of things you do not really need. When it comes to finding out what it is that is setting you off and how intense the reaction is, you need something which is ready to hand and easy to read when reviewing at the end of the week/month. I believe that recording your urticaria is essential in beating it. Over months you might suddenly feel much better, but why? What changed? With recorded data you can look back and notice what changed for you so you know that if times get bad again you can revert to what worked before. I record my data using two methods. One easy statistical measure, for daily itching/weals on a spreadsheet, and an attack diary of just a single line describing the situation and previous food consumption/exercise.

I recommend recording both what you were doing at the time of an attack, and what you have eaten / drank most recently that day. For this, just a simple notepad is need, but if you have a smart phone download Wunderlist (Available on Android, iOS, Windows Phone and desktop) or a similar to do list app. You probably always have your phone on you, so it is there and ready to make any notes of what happened while it is fresh in your mind. I also like Wunderlist as it has a desktop app for Windows/Mac that syncs to your phone/tablet so you can literally update it anywhere. Plus its basic version is free. Once setup, create a new list for attacks, write down what happened as and when, and you will start to see a pattern(s) over time.

Just keep it simple and write about the following:

- Most recent food and drink
- What activity specifically set you off
- Temperature and temperature change if applicable
- Any variations like, particularly bad hives, last longer than normal?

Some actual examples from my food diary

- Walking around in and out of shops, coldish day, bacon sandwich hours before
- Curry towards end of meal (not spicy), at home, room fairly warm

- Same day as Cycling, after food (Burger), going into warm pub, climbed steep hill

As you can see it doesn't matter how you write it, just needs to be in a way you can understand it

The next step is to measure your itching and its intensity so you can follow your progress. Bare in mind that most changes you do will not be instant, so you need to track over days, sometimes weeks to see what has made the difference. I modified an assessment chart that I was given to show this (see next page).

	M	T	W	T	F	S	S	M	T	W	T	F	S	S
Date Started														
Notes														
	M	T	W	T	F	S	S	M	T	W	T	F	S	S
WEALS														
None (0)														
< 20 Small (1)														
20-50 Small (2)														
>50 or Large (3)														
Score (0-3)														
	M	T	W	T	F	S	S	M	T	W	T	F	S	S
ITCHING														
None (0)														
Mild (1)														
Moderate (2)														
Intense (3)														
Score (0-3)														
Daily Total (0-6)														
Weekly Total (0-42)														

The chart is very simple to fill in. Just put crosses in the section that relates to you on that day. You can do it at the end of the day, or if you have had a maximum attack just fill it in afterwards. In the notes section, just write what you have done/tried/changed. i.e. if you have changed medication or did a good workout. You could even write down a brief pointer on what it was that set you off to rate intensity to foods etc. You don't need to do the notes everyday though. If you start different antihistamine tablets on a Tuesday just write it down once until you change to something else. But note down if you missed a day, increased dosage or stopped etc. Likewise if you go to acupuncture or start a new type of diet then note this down. Hopefully once you start getting a hold of this you will see a pattern of your score getting lower, and that is a great feeling to look back at where you have come from, especially on the bad days.

Ways to Help When The Itching Comes

One of the biggest questions asked is what can you do once the itching has arrived, bar popping a pill. Over the years I have tried several different techniques, which I'm sure many of you have your own, but here is what works for me with a rudimentary rating on its effectiveness and difficulty. **Side note, if you are driving or operating something dangerous, stop, pull over in a safe spot. Never try to work through itching while doing something which requires concentration.**

AVOID THAT FIRST SCRATCH
Difficulty 5/5
Effectiveness 4/5
Easy to say, incredibly difficult to do. But if you can do it, you will lose the hives and itching quicker than any other method. However small that first scratch is we all know what will come next is more scratching, itching and pain. It is simple to write this off as impossible but I have done it on several occasions and you get such an amazing feeling when you do it. Count to ten in your head, try and notice everything around you in the tiniest detail, concentrate on your breathing. Do whatever you can to take your mind off it. If you can stop your hands from raising to your head or arm, and hold it for 30 seconds to a minute you can get over the worst part and you feel this rush as the itching peaks and drops off. Some people prefer to clear the mind, I try to fill it with crazy detail. Try it, it will not be possible every time, and for me very rarely at the beginning, but the reward is an incredible feeling of satisfaction. Another technique you can use to help this is...

THE HAND CLENCH
Difficulty 4/5
Effectiveness 4/5
The itching is in full swing, you cannot take it anymore you have to scratch, what can you do as a last ditch effort to try and avoid scratching... Clench your fist tight! Do not let go until its gone. Another tough one, but again it can be very effective. The downside to this, its hard to maintain a train of

thought while doing this. You can only really do it while standing or seating not doing anything with your hands. A good modification to this is to grab your leg through your trouser pockets. Again its all about removing the focus from the trigger area to somewhere else. Grabbing your leg can be subtle, and very effective working in a similar way to the hand clench. Do not pinch the skin but squeeze and hold your muscle with an open palm. The difficulty here is holding out when the itching gets very bad, because if like me your arms get very bad regularly, when your arms are tense, as they will be doing this, it can effect the outbreak.

WEAR LONG SLEEVES

Difficulty 1/5

Effectiveness 3/5

This is all about ease of access. Ever seen a dog with a lampshade or a child with mittens to stop them scratching their skin? Well this is a less extreme version of this. If you are in a t-shirt and can see the hives coming up, it makes your mind want to do nothing but scratch that itch. But by also putting on a top that covers the common itchy areas you can make it that little bit harder to scratch. Obviously lifting a t-shirt is not difficult, but its a mental barrier which can make a difference, similar to how studies have shown having a small fence reduces your chance of robbery. It's not about ultimate protect, just enough for the brain to think otherwise. As a side note, when cycling, I found wearing a long sleeve top reduced arm flare ups even in hot weather vs a normal t-shirt. So even though I was hotter, and the wind could not cool me down I got less attacks. In winter wear gloves for the same reason.

WEAR MORE CLOTHES DURING EXERCISE

Difficulty 1/5 but 5/5 to make effective

Effectiveness 4/5

Somewhat related to the previous point, but an important one. As you know, my itching when exercising comes just before I was about to sweat. However once I managed to work through it and because I was exercising hard, I started sweating, as you do. Within around 30 seconds I noticed the itching was gone. So next time I tried to make myself warm from the beginning. Now you may want to do this at home, rather than at the gym as it will get some looks. I wore a hooded sweater, hat, gloves and additional trousers over my shorts while doing a workout. I looked and felt a fool, however it made me perspire much quicker than normal, which allowed me to get over the itching phase. The only problem, was the initial itching was horrendous. The only thing that stopped me was gripping extremely hard (hand clench) and the fact I had so many layers on my skin was all covered. However once it did not last nearly as long as normal, and once gone the feeling was bliss. Do not try this in a gym please you will look like a crazy person, and if at home make sure someone is about to make sure you are ok as you may get very hot. Drink lots of water! In fact I would recommend you all increase your water intake. Nothing hydrates and flushes out your body like water.

PRE-EMPTIVELY DEAL WITH IT
Difficulty 3/5
Effectiveness 4/5 (With Practise)
You are likely to have an attack, but that is OK and we will deal with it as it comes. If you can get that simple statement into your head you will have less and milder flare ups. I noticed this after accepting my "fate" a couple of times and not having such a bad attack or not at all. It is all about changing of your mind set. As an example, previously you go into a restaurant and think, "its warm in here, there are a lot of people... when is it going to happen, OK its happening!" But with this in mind, change your mind set before you leave you think, "OK, I'm going to a restaurant, there will be trigger foods, I will avoid the food with chilis however much I want them, the restaurant will be busy and probably warm so I will remove coats etc as soon as I get in, and go to the toilet to acclimatise to the situation. We will ask for a table in a well vented spot. If that is not possible I will deal with the itching when it comes. I'm just going to have a great time with friends" It is not about being negative, but by preparing yourself for possible outcomes so you have no worries when (if) the itching comes. I have found at worst by trusting this mindset has reduced itching to a minor inconvenience to fully enjoying a meal without any thought of itching.

Going shopping? Do the same, run the likely scenarios in your head. You know they will have the heating on full blast so the staff can be in t-shirts in December, so do not get angry and anxious about it. Prepare and think ahead, knowing you can deal with it if such a moment occurs.

I know this is easy to say but harder to do in practise. There will always be situations you could not of planned for, but if you can think through a lot of them, you will be in a good frame of mind that you can enjoy your outing, and you will not think about urticaria as much anyway. Being in a positive frame of mind is one of the most overlooked ways to improve urticaria, probably because there is no black and white way of measuring it. I have no doubts that having urticaria destroys self esteem and your confidence around people. This is far beyond the scope of this book, however I would recommend reading or watching videos on people like Tony Robbins and Eric Thomas. They specialise on improving your inner self.

Urticaria will reduce your confidence, and it can be hard to find a place to start building it back up. One of the biggest mistakes people make is they want confidence but don't know what that means to them. Confidence is not a metric scale. It is something only you can decide, to one person it might mean something completely different to someone else. To one person being confident is being able to stand up in front of 1000 people and do a speech. To another guy its being able to step outside his house and go to the shops without fear. The only way you can have confidence is by defining what it means to have confidence for you and then working out how you can gain those traits one by one. If you feel urticaria has shot your confidence then ask yourself what would it be like to be the ideal you, where urticaria does not bother you and you have supreme confidence to do anything. Then work out some small gains, such as setting your self a goal each day that is achievable. For example the way I did with my cycling. Small loops, getting bigger each outing. Keep building on it but have no zero days. Make sure you always do at least one thing a day, whether its one press up, one sentence, anything! Record it and within a few weeks you can look back with pride at what you have achieved. For more on this check out Reddit r/NoZeroDay and r/DecidingToBeBetter. Like urticaria, confidence is something which you can build on bit by bit and before it you have positive results, and you can get your life back.

www.ingramcontent.com/pod-product-compliance
Lightning Source LLC
Chambersburg PA
CBHW021407160726
47994CB00007B/3112